# The Eye of the

# Storm

## The Silent Grief of Miscarriage

Rachel McGrath

# DEDICATION

Dedicated to the many brave strong women who have faced the loss of miscarriage, and to those family, friends and loved ones who have supported me through my pain.

# THE FOREWORD

Losing someone you love is heartbreaking, but what if you never had a chance to hold the one you loved in person?

Pregnancy loss is a tragedy that affects many women, but sadly, it is seldom spoken of openly. In fact, for many women who experience early pregnancy loss in their first trimester, it is hardly even noticed. Some argue that it was not yet a fully formed fetus, measuring only millimeters in length. Yet, despite the physical form, that pregnancy still remains a lost hope of motherhood, and with the passing of that small life inside, it brings grief and pain that perhaps will never be forgotten, no matter what the future brings.

As someone who has felt the pain of miscarriage, I wonder why we feel the need to hide such a loss and silently grieve for a baby that could never be. I don't believe that there is an absolute right or wrong way of dealing with such a loss. Yet, I found that there was a sense of discomfort and sometimes awkwardness when sharing my news, seeking solace or a compassionate ear to talk to. At times, I felt that by talking about my miscarriage, I was upsetting the social norm, and my struggles with trying to conceive and carry a baby created more of an imposition on others who perhaps did not fully understand my dilemma.

At times there seemed to be an expectation that I would recover quickly, move on, that perhaps it wasn't a real loss, such as the death of a relative. Many seemed to misunderstand the anxiety and torment that miscarriage leaves with you; you never forget the pain, and it lingers through future pregnancies, as you fear that the same will happen again. There have been countless times, where others have offered me solutions to *solve* my fear of miscarriage or my inability to carry a child: IVF, adoption, surrogacy. Alas, when you lose a loved one, you don't suddenly seek options to replace them; you just want to grieve. That is the real misunderstanding with early pregnancy loss. We all need time to grieve.

The sympathy of friends and family certainly came to us in abundance as we dealt openly with our early pregnancy losses. But, still there were times when it was expected that all was well, and I would carry on with life as normal, that the past was in the past. It was during those moments when I felt the most alone with my grief and misfortune. Writing about my feelings and pain throughout this time helped me, giving me a personal solace through the expression of my experiences in words on paper.

My one hope in publishing this short memoir is to release my pain and ultimately support and connect with other women who have also experienced the pain and grief of early pregnancy loss; perhaps there is comfort in knowing that we are not alone.

Each and every situation is different; my experiences are my own, and through this story I have written my deep intimate thoughts, my insanity and my personal experience through the loss of a child that I would never hold. I offer no advice and I am not a medical expert on this subject. I seek nothing more than to share my journey with others.

## THE PAIN

     I paced impatiently back and forth across the small waiting room. I couldn't sit down. I had been here before, and those memories of the last time reinforced my growing anxiety. It was the not knowing, that daunting feeling that we were about to receive bad news yet again; the waiting was torturous. I had a growing urge to scream out loud or just cry. *Hurry up!* I prayed to myself; I felt like this waiting was literally driving me insane.

The rational side of me could see clearly that there were others in front of me. I was probably irritating them with my obvious anxiety. They were undoubtedly feeling exactly the same way, just hiding it better. At this moment in time, all that I could think about was what I was about to find out in that little room; any time now. This moment had been in my every waking thought for over two weeks since I first booked the appointment. *Is this pregnancy the one?*

I truly despised this place. Sad, tragic memories flooded me as I recalled the last time I had entered that little ultrasound room. Déjà vu overwhelmed me as I mentally played out the events of last time and wondered whether I would again walk away heartbroken. Surely, it could not happen again. This time had to be different; I wasn't sure how I could face any more bad news. I forced myself to quietly assure myself this time it would be a positive result, despite all of the anxieties running rife inside of me. *This time has to be our time!*

In many ways, my pulse was jumping with the increasing anticipation, hoping with every morsel of my heart for good news, but in readiness to hear the worst yet again.

Why did I put myself through this? Well, there was one very good reason: the only reason. My greatest desire has always been to become a mother!

I was six weeks and five days pregnant, to be perfectly exact. I had been pregnant before, but alas, I still had no children, just little angels that never made it to my seventh week of pregnancy. I had been here before, to this point, and never made it further. That is why this day was so very important; it was the milestone we needed to pass, the point we had reached with every other pregnancy but never been able to journey beyond. *Today has to be different. Today, I hope to see a heartbeat!*

The loss and heartache of miscarriage is something that is so very real to many women, yet it is a world that is mostly hidden in silent grief. I had experienced that grief far too much, and in many ways, I was still raw from the hurt of past losses. Yet I kept returning for more, hoping that destiny or Mother Nature would lend me a helping hand this time, allowing this next pregnancy to prevail. That was my one and only hope.

I stopped pacing for a moment in front of my husband. He looked up at me and sighed. He was nervous, and I was frustrating him with my impatience. Whilst he told me that he was confident this time, his eyes told me a different story. In many ways, I felt as though we were preparing ourselves for another fall. He nodded to the seat beside him, and obligingly, I took a seat. He reached across and took my hand, and as his thumb traced circles on my palm, I felt comforted by his presence and his strength. I would not have survived this far without him. I looked into his eyes and smiled. No matter what the outcome, we had each other.

After what seemed to be an eternity of waiting and just watching other couples going in and out of that little door leading to the small, dark ultrasound room, our name was finally called. I felt my husband's hand give mine a small, tight squeeze. We looked at each other and smiled nervously before standing up to follow the nurse into the small room.

Unfortunately, I knew this procedure all too well. As the curtain was pulled for my privacy, I prepared myself, removing my trousers and seating myself on the small bed right next to the monitor. I looked at the tiny monitor right beside the bed hopefully. In just a few moments, that small screen would reveal the fate of our pregnancy. *Just breathe,* I remind myself as the anxiousness started to rise up.

I leant back against the small pillow and called out to the nurse that I was ready to start.

The curtain was drawn, and my husband followed behind her, giving me a reassuring smile. *Here goes,* I sighed deeply, praying that in the next few minutes we would get the assurance that my heart most desired, a strong, healthy heartbeat and a growing pregnancy.

The silence in the room suddenly felt deafening as my eyes moved back and forth from the nurse and then to my husband, playing Ping-Pong between the two. I was desperately trying to read their separate expressions. My husband was watching the monitor intently. I wondered if he could see anything, and whether he even understood what he was seeing. I couldn't tell; his face seemed unreadable. I moved my gaze to the nurse and watched expectantly as I felt her wiggle the ultrasound wand into position, her eyes transfixed on the monitor. She didn't speak, just kept clicking buttons on the machine in front her. From my own position, I couldn't see the monitor screen, so I had no way of even getting a hint of good or bad news. I gave up trying to read her expression and lay back against the pillow, closing my eyes and just waiting for someone to break the silence. Seconds felt like hours as I waited, and then she spoke.

"I am so sorry!" Those four little words suddenly shattered everything inside of me. I thought I could hear my heart break in that moment. I sat upright in shock and swiveled around to see the monitor. I could see something, but I wasn't sure what I should be looking for. I looked back at her, my eyes already filling with tears as I hoped I had heard wrong. The nurse merely shook her head sadly. "I can see the gestational sac and a small foetus, but there is no heartbeat. It's dating over a week behind. I'm sorry, your pregnancy has stopped."

I looked at my husband, who took my hand and rubbed it softly. We had been here before, but we still weren't fully prepared to hear those words again. My husband didn't say a word, but I knew he was heartbroken. I couldn't hold in the tears as the pain became unbearable.

The nurse took the hint to give us some space. "Please take your time to get dressed and then we can talk?" She probably saw this often, but her empathy was obvious. She quietly put the equipment away, turned and pulled the curtain closed behind her, allowing me to dress. My husband leant over and kissed me gently on the forehead. This felt like a bad recurring nightmare, and I couldn't believe we were reliving it again. I wanted to just lie there, curl up into a ball and forget the world around me. It was my husband who reached to squeeze my shoulder, hinting that I needed to get dressed.

I sat up and shifted off the bed, getting re-dressed as though I was on autopilot, quietly sobbing, knowing that the worst was yet to come. I couldn't believe we were here again, and it was the same as last time; no heartbeat. I couldn't fathom how I would survive it this time. I had only just recovered from the last miscarriage. This pregnancy had been our renewed hope. Now that hope was gone as well.

Finally dressed, I sat beside the nurse, my husband standing next to me, his hand resting on my shoulder in support. I half-listened as the nurse gently explained that the fetus was dating at around five weeks, that it had not developed to where it should have. I was told that I should expect to start miscarrying naturally in the coming week, as the gestational sac was misshapen, showing that the pregnancy had ended over a week ago.

It was her job, but it all sounded so clinical. All I could think was that my baby was dead inside of me for over a week. My hand touched my stomach, as though I was comforting the small fetus inside of me that had passed. He or she, I would never know which, was gone, and now I had to wait for my body to let it go. It was all too overwhelming.

Our last miscarriage was only six months

ago. I had only just recovered physically when I found out we were pregnant again. I thought this was another chance, fate's way of giving us back the hope we had lost. Perhaps I should have been more prepared this time, but I wasn't sure you could really prepare for anything like this.

After what seemed an overload of tests and information, my husband and I finally left the hospital. We walked to our car hand-in-hand, in silence. As we drove home, we spoke of small, inconsequential topics to break the intense silence and the grief that we were feeling. It was easier to discuss whether we would call in sick for work, or whether we wanted to pick up some bread for lunch, rather than really talk about the fact that we had lost another pregnancy. The reality was all too real and raw for either of us to face head-on at that moment in time.

## THE FEELING

As we stepped through the front door of our home, our small dog greeted us enthusiastically. For a brief moment, I forgot about what had just happened, and I bent down to give the excited pup a scratch between the ears. It was a welcome distraction as he inclined his head towards my hand, seeking more attention and scratches.

The moment was brief and my reprieve

dissipated as reality came crashing back, and the pain intensified once more. I stood upright, and my husband and I just looked at each other sadly. He held out his arms, and I moved in to hold him. I didn't want to let go; the comfort of my husband's strong arms felt like the protection I needed from the myriad of battered feelings that felt like they were brimming on the edge of just losing it. I wanted to scream, but I didn't have the strength to even whisper.

The entire situation felt completely surreal. Only a few hours ago, we had left this house, our hopes raised with anticipation that this time all would be okay. Returning home, everything had suddenly changed, and yet physically I still felt the same. I still felt pregnant.

I wandered aimlessly around the house for a while. I didn't know what to do with myself. Emotionally, I felt numb; physically, I felt absolutely fine. I didn't want to lie down; I couldn't relax. I needed to keep myself occupied, take my mind off the hurt, but I didn't know what I could do. I was lost inside my own home.

"Tea?" My husband offered. I nodded and smiled weakly at him, grateful. *I should sit and watch a movie*, I thought to myself. But I knew I wouldn't sit still, and whatever I did to try to distract myself, I knew it wouldn't work. I couldn't shake the fact that I had lost my baby today, replaying out the events in that small ultrasound room over and over again.

I remembered feeling the same way before, and those feelings resurfaced again. I didn't know how I should be reacting right then. I wanted to cry and curl up in a ball, but instead I ended up just sitting in silence in my living room, staring at the blank screen of our television. My hands kept touching my stomach, knowing that what was in there was no longer alive and growing. That alone seemed to be the most difficult concept for me to fathom. Only millimeters in size, that small being was gone, but it was still there, not yet departed.

My body had not yet shown any signs of changes through the early weeks of this pregnancy. I had a little bit of bloating, but the average person would never have been able to tell that I was just over six weeks pregnant. For me, however, I had changed over the past weeks. There had been an excitement building inside of me with the promise of a new life growing and my hopes of becoming a mother. Now that was all gone.

A steaming cup of tea was placed on the small coffee table in front of me, and my husband sat silently beside me, placing his strong arm around my waist. I turned to him and we hugged. Whilst we didn't talk about it, I felt comforted knowing that I had him by my side, and whilst I felt I was falling apart, he seemed to have the strength I needed at that moment to pick up the pieces. We were both hurting, grieving this loss, albeit in different ways.

As I held him, I wondered how he could be so strong. I knew he was hurting too, but I would never understand how this loss truly touched him. He was there from the first moment, when I had come running out of the bathroom with the positive pregnancy test; he had joined my elation when we realised we were pregnant again. Then, as the anxiety and paranoia started through those first few weeks of pregnancy, he had calmed my fears, encouraging me to stay positive. Above everything, I knew that I had his strength and support when I felt like I was falling apart. I was grateful to have him here, just holding me as I dwelled in the sadness of the news we heard just hours ago. It felt like our quest to become parents was moving further from our reach and that Mother Nature was working against us.

I received a text asking how the scan went, and I hesitated before replying. We had told only a few close family and friends, and they had been excited, hopeful and anxious, as we had been, about this pregnancy. Now I just wanted to hide from the world for this one moment in time. I didn't want to interact with anyone but my husband. We were both experiencing this firsthand, and I didn't feel like anyone else could truly help us through the pain. The more I thought about, the more I felt myself crumble under the grief. My mind was whirring with thoughts of what if, what next, what now. My heart felt heavy, my head hurt with the loss, and my body was crying the tears that had stopped falling from my eyes.

This feeling was like nothing else I had ever experienced, not even through the death of loved ones, heartbreak, or even failure. I couldn't describe the emotions that were spinning around inside of me. It was as though my own body had betrayed me, that this lifelong promise of becoming a mother and starting a family had all been a lie. I felt cheated by Mother Nature, and that moment in that small ultrasound room, where we had placed all of our hopes, had been taken away from us with no remorse. It felt unfair.

# *THE MORNING AFTER*

After struggling to fall asleep that first night after our news, my body finally gave into exhaustion, and I was able to sleep for a few hours at least. Waking early the next morning, there was a moment where I forgot the events of the day before. Over the past few weeks, I had woken each morning with the thought that it was one day further in my pregnancy, and on this morning, I had momentarily reverted back to that feeling. But that moment was fleeting, as my oblivion passed and my sleep-induced memory re-triggered the events of the day before. My pregnancy was over.

Even though I knew the baby was gone, my body was still sending pregnancy signals. My breasts were slightly tender and my body felt lethargic. I knew this was the pregnancy hormone, which was still active in my body, playing tricks with my mind and invoking foolish thoughts that the nurse had made some drastic error. The sensible side of me knew this wasn't possible, but the grieving part of me struggled to let go. Alas, no miracle was going to reverse time. I slumped back into my pillow and closed my eyes, knowing that today was going to offer me nothing more, and now was just a waiting game for my body to release this lost pregnancy.

*How do I move on from here?* The same question circled around my thoughts. I had survived this before, but in some ways I had reconciled that loss as perhaps my body's way of reacting to a first pregnancy. I had been told that one in four pregnancies end in a miscarriage, and I had told myself that the next time would be our time for sure. How I had been so very wrong!

I didn't want to get out of bed; I didn't want to face any reality, but I knew that I couldn't hide forever. Forcing myself to have a shower, I went to the bathroom expecting to find some signs of this miscarriage. Nothing. I felt like I was merely waiting for the process to start. In some ways, I hoped it would start soon, and I strangely wanted to feel the physically pain, so that I could feel something real.

I remembered last time I lost my pregnancy at just over six weeks. I found at the time, many understood that we were hurting, yet because nothing had changed physically, the loss wasn't visible. It wasn't until I felt the physical effects of the miscarriage that even I truly accepted the loss. When it did finally happen, I kept forcing myself to think of it as a really heavy menstrual cycle, that the past six weeks had been almost a delusion. In some ways, aside from the emotional grief, many could have assumed that I was actually fine. Perhaps that was what I wanted them to think. But, alas, I certainly didn't feel "fine."

The morning after should have been a workday, but the thought of walking through those office doors was completely unfathomable. I couldn't just pretend that everything was normal, and there was no way I could focus on the job at hand when all of my insides felt like they were screaming to be heard. My colleagues had no idea; I hadn't told them I was pregnant, so they would never realise the turmoil of the loss I was now experiencing. Today was not any other day. It wasn't the same; I couldn't pretend that I was okay, not today, perhaps not even tomorrow.

Showered and dressed, I decided that the only place I wanted to be was inside my bed. So

I decided to indulge myself as I climbed back under the covers and curled my body tightly into a ball, burying myself underneath the sheets and blankets and hoping I could sleep just a little bit longer and forget everything for a while. I wanted it all to go away, but unfortunately, my mind continued to race with thoughts of self-pity and hurt.

My husband was still in bed too, although I could sense he was awake. Neither of us spoke. He rolled over and moved in closer to me, wrapping his arms around me. It was the comfort I needed, the silent affection that told me he was feeling the pain too. As I lay there in his arms, I wondered if we would ever be parents? I was afraid of what the future may look like, and even the thought of trying again was daunting. It was too early, and we couldn't really answer these questions just yet, but I did start to wonder how many losses we could endure as a couple. I certainly never wanted to feel this way again, but I also couldn't control

Mother Nature.

We agreed to take the day off from work and spend time together. Technically neither of us could be counted as unwell, but we were both grieving a loss. Perhaps to some the grief wasn't obvious; there was no funeral, no ceremony, and we could not celebrate a life that had not been lived. Our baby had not even seen the light of day. Some could say that it was too early to even be called a baby, but it was still a life. A life that had been growing inside of me; and it was still in there, but the life itself was gone.

We hadn't made any plans for the day; we just wanted to spend it together, being there for each other. We decided to get out of the house, have lunch somewhere locally and face the real world. It was as we were about to leave the house when a deep, painful cramp ran through my stomach. I stopped, held my lower abdomen and let the pain pulse through me until it eased slightly. This was my first real physical sign that the miscarriage was about to begin.

That first cramp only lasted for less than a minute, but it quickly removed any delusions about the day before; this was real, and it was happening, again. Now I only hoped that it would all be short and painless and over with quickly, so I could really move on.

# *THE OTHERS*

I felt like I was falling apart with grief and sadness inside, yet all around me, no one was aware of what I was really going through. As I walked down the street or entered my local store, nobody knew that I was miscarrying. Aside from my own pain, there were no obvious visible signs. I looked no different than I did a few days earlier, only perhaps lacking the excitement and obvious thrill of actually being pregnant. In the harsh light of day, the fact that I was miscarrying was completely invisible to the public eye.

It was such a lonely place to be right then. Of course I had my husband by my side, and he was ever supportive and caring. Nonetheless, we were alone. We didn't walk down the street and open up the conversation with our situation. It felt as though no one could truly grasp what I was feeling, and the sadness that overwhelmed me was somewhat off-putting in general conversation. So I didn't speak about it. I pretended all was okay; I was surviving and we would move on. But in truth, the thought of moving on was difficult.

There have been times when I just wanted to scream, shout, cry out loud; sometimes I wanted to tell people that I was miserable, that I was losing my baby, and I just couldn't cope with the pain. Yet, I just couldn't. It wasn't done. The general expectation was that you do carry on, console yourself with those closest around you and hope that all will be okay. However, at that very moment, it really was not okay.

As we were seated in the restaurant, a young waitress enthusiastically handed us our menus. "How are you today?" she asked lightly. I smiled feebly at her, focusing on opening up the menu and attempting to avoid the answer.

"Good, thanks," my husband answered politely on my behalf. I looked up from behind the menu, sending him a brief thank you with just my eyes.

"Any drinks to start?" she asked, oblivious to my melancholy mood.

"Just give us a moment, thanks," he said kindly to her but clearly sending her a signal that we wanted some space to talk and perhaps decide on our meal.

"No problem, I'll be back shortly," her voice practically sang, and in many ways I was grateful for her energy; I needed it to bring me back to the real world.

"Would you like a glass of wine?" My husband asked me as she walked away. I looked at him blankly and then realised. *Oh yes, I had been abstaining from all alcohol during the pregnancy. However, now, technically, I could drink,* I thought to myself. *But do I want to drink?* It somehow felt strange, as until now I had been focused on eating all the right things and avoiding all food and drinks that were on the non-advisory list for pregnant women. Another strong cramp hit my stomach, like a sign reminding me that this pregnancy was gone, and perhaps reinforcing that I was now free to eat and drink what I pleased. That thought itself renewed the sadness that we were being forced to start again; like the pregnancy never really happened.

"Yes," I heard myself say without even thinking. "A white wine, please." I needed to give myself something today. As I read through the menu, I decided on the pâté as a starter. *Why not?* I told myself; I deserved to give myself something I could try to enjoy. In a strange way, this was my small way of confirming to myself that this was not just a bad dream; it was a reality, and I had to face the future knowing that I would not be holding a newborn baby in less than nine months' time.

As we sat eating our lunch, I couldn't help but look around the small restaurant. There were many couples, friends, and groups of people eating. It made me wonder what their story was. Perhaps someone else in this room, like me, was experiencing some sort of pain or grief as well. As I glanced at each table, I tried to read any signals that would lead me to believe my theory was true. However, like me, on the outside, all seemed normal and okay.

Selfishly, I needed to believe that perhaps someone within that small dining room would understand my grief if I were to tell them. In a strange way, it helped me to reconcile that I was not truly alone, that there were others out there like me. That this overwhelming grief I was feeling was actually normal. That the sadness would dissipate eventually, and perhaps one day in the future, we may consider trying again.

But for now, I would concentrate on trying to enjoy the glass of wine and eating a real meal. Today, I would focus on *acting* normal in public.

# *THE GRIEF*

Sure enough, within the next twenty-four hours I started to bleed. It was heavier than a period and more painful, but I had experienced this before. I had known in some ways what I should expect. Still, it didn't feel any easier this time around.

In a strange way, however, it felt as though the physical pain I was experiencing reinforced the emotional hurt that surrounded my every waking thought. At times, I found myself embracing the excruciating ache inside my abdomen and the pulsing cramps; sometimes I even avoided taking the pain medications that would have eased the pain substantially. Why? Bizarrely, the pain allowed me to tangibly feel this loss, and as I lay there crying, I felt like it reinforced the hurt that was haunting my thoughts, and the grief itself felt more real.

The worst of it lasted for around five days, and whilst I did not go into the office, I allowed myself to work from home. I was not yet ready to face the real world but knew I couldn't hide behind my own four walls forever. Many of my colleagues would just assume that I was unwell; I lied, saying that I had contracted a stomach virus. I used that as the excuse, as it generally didn't raise too many questions. In a way, it was a legitimate excuse; something inside of me had stopped the growth of my pregnancy, perhaps that virus was me?

The unfortunate truth was that regardless of the excuse, my colleagues had not been aware of my pregnancy, and when I finally did return to work, they would never know any different. They would ask how I was feeling, as though I was recovering from a standard "bug," and I wondered how I would respond and whether things would feel better with time.

On the several calls I attended remotely from my bed, I did have questions from my colleagues, polite enquiries on my health, and brief "get well soon" encouragements. Over the phone, it felt easier to answer questions without going into detail. I would quickly defer the conversation back to work, and no one was the wiser at my unease with their empathetic questions. In many ways, sitting on calls helped to refocus my mind onto other matters, and I found myself turning off from my own pain momentarily, helping to remind me that life really does go on.

We didn't have a ceremony or any event

that would signify the remembrance of our little lost angel. Perhaps we should have? That in itself was a quandary for me. I had seen many other women in my position purchase something that would provide that remembrance. Truth be told, I didn't know what I could buy to really signify the loss I was feeling. Nothing in my mind could quantify this grief.

We all cope differently, and for me, I needed my husband by my side during this time; that was all. As a couple, we spoke about what we needed from each other; we made plans to spend time together—a weekend away, a night out at the movies, and sometimes, it was a home-cooked meal and a quiet night on the sofa.

Over the days that progressed, I found myself slowly accepting the fate of this pregnancy, and my bouts of tears seemed less frequent with each day. Nevertheless, the hurt and grief itself didn't fade. Whilst I understood that we were back to square one on this conception journey, there was still the regret of what could never be that haunted my thoughts.

During a previous miscarriage, in an attempt to provide consolation, I was told that when I finally have my healthy baby I would forget all the pain and grief, and it would all be worth it. I couldn't ever imagine forgetting, and I didn't want to. If and when I was finally able to conceive a healthy baby, I would remember all the angels we lost and knew that in some way, they would always be with me. I had to believe that, or this pain I was feeling now was all for nothing. Truly, however, the grief never leaves; it just becomes manageable.

# *THE REALITY*

As they say, *life goes on.*

The first real day back at work, in the office, I knew would be difficult. It had been before, and it would be again. I recalled the last time I had been here like it was déjà vu. As I entered my office building, everything at the time had felt surreal, and I remembered standing in the foyer like a lost lamb, unsure of how I would even walk to my office, let alone make it through the next eight hours. As my colleagues offered friendly greetings, welcoming me back to work, I had run for solace inside the bathroom cubicle. At that time, I felt cheated by everything, ashamed that I could not face the real world, and ready to shut myself away and avoid all human contact.

This time around, it felt no easier. I wasn't sure if I had expected it to be, or not, but again I felt the walls of my car closing in on me as I pulled into the office carpark. Every emotion from the past week swept through me as I sat in my stationary car outside the entrance to my office building. I couldn't even bring myself to turn off the engine and just stared numbly at the big brown building looming in front of me.

There was no reason why I could not work today; physically, I was no longer in pain. Regardless, my motivation and mood could not fathom the idea of trivial small talk or office banter, nor did I feel any interest for the priorities of my business. Nothing made any sense to me when I felt I had lost so much personally.

As I finally plucked up the courage to exit my vehicle and enter the office, the effort of walking itself became a chore, and I did all I could to stop myself from crying. For some reason, the acceptance that I had started to feel about my situation now felt like it was spinning into reverse. I wanted to go back home and curl up under my blanket. However, I needed to force myself to move forward, and I had come this far. I kept reminding myself that I just had to get through this one day, and hopefully it would slowly get easier.

For the first part of the morning, I kept my office door closed, happy enough to avoid the real world but feeling as though I had made progress by physically being at work. It was easier to pretend I was still in my solitary bubble if I didn't have to speak to people, but I knew that would not last for very long. My job was not a solo role; I had to talk to people, and I could not avoid the inevitable.

I had a mid-morning meeting, and deciding to emerge from my bubble, I braved the boardroom where many of my colleagues congregated. I found it fairly easy to become absorbed into the project meeting agenda, and for a moment, I felt like a normal human being again. However, that was short-lived when the meeting adjourned, and general conversation took place.

I found it exhausting as I tried to avoid personal and social topics of conversation. Each time, they seemed to naturally veer to family life, social outings, children, holidays; the trivial matters that seemed so inconsequential to me at this point in time. It was all unavoidable, however, especially because to all who were outside of my world, those were just general topics that surround normal conversation. Only, to me, nothing felt normal that day.

At lunchtime, I stood in the queue waiting to be served and felt myself freeze as I noticed the woman waiting next to me. She held her back as her beautiful round pregnancy bump shifted into my view. I couldn't help but look at it with envy, as she unconsciously rubbed her belly. I estimated that she must have been at least six or seven months pregnant. I felt a pang of jealousy as I longed for this woman's joy; I was once again reminded of what I wouldn't experience in the months to come. It took all of my strength just to maintain my composure and get through the rest of the day.

It was all a process, and with each setback, I had to force myself to keep moving forward, not to stop and get caught up in the pain. When I felt that I was hitting a roadblock, I would tell myself that this constant hurt would slowly subside, that with time, I would feel normal again.

# THE WORDS

I wasn't sure that there really is an exact "right thing to say" to any woman who has recently miscarried her pregnancy.

Nothing could really comfort or heal the pain and grief I was experiencing. Whilst I felt grateful for the empathy and support others gave me, it was all just words to me and it still left me standing alone and suffering. We had only chosen to share the news of our pregnancy with close family and friends. In hindsight, perhaps we should have kept it completely private, but we were so excited at the time, and we were bursting to share our joy! Those who we did tell knew our full history with miscarriage, and perhaps naively I had believed the odds were in our favour this time.

Did I regret it? Not really. Those first few weeks of pregnancy were so difficult and stressful, it was sometimes comforting to share those anxieties with loved ones. Sometimes, all I needed was a little bit of reassurance or sound advice from those around me. More importantly, I needed allies. There were times when keeping my early pregnancy a secret was extremely difficult. Colleagues at work and other friends would quickly notice small changes in behaviour, and I certainly didn't want to face any questions when I didn't know myself, for sure, whether this pregnancy would last to full term. Having a select few who knew of my condition allowed me some release and sometimes backup when I needed to find creative ways to disclose my condition.

Essentially, I would never regret telling our close friends and family; it was the right thing to do at the time. However, the true difficulty came when we had to tell them, one by one, that the pregnancy had failed. It was hard; first, because I was only just dealing with my sorrow, and then having to deal with the reactions of others unwittingly exacerbated that pain. It was challenging for everyone. I could tell that some of our loved ones struggled with what to say or how to offer sympathy. But, really, that was understandable. Whilst some had been in our position before, perhaps in different ways, others hadn't and could only imagine what we were experiencing. The entire ordeal was difficult and emotional, and rightly or wrongly, I had put them in that position.

There were no words that could make everything all better. Oddly, I found myself getting upset as words of condolence were offered but failed to provide the compassion and healing I was seeking to make me feel better. They were just words, and words would not bring back what I had lost.

As I was experiencing this roller coaster of emotions, it was easy enough to find fault in anything, to become impatient with the world around me. I felt cheated by the entire process, and I needed something or someone to get angry at. Yet, I had to remind myself that the words of support we were receiving were made in good faith, and to be honest, I wasn't sure what I could say myself to someone else in my own position.

Even now, having experienced miscarriage firsthand and knowing the pain and hurt that I have felt, it is difficult to truly comprehend the myriad of emotions or needs that you succumb to at the lowest point of your grief. Whilst I had become more sensitive to the seemingly right or wrong things to say, I understood that everyone is different. The cycle of emotions I had experienced since finding out that my pregnancy failed was constantly interchangeable and unpredictable.

Just as there were moments when I felt I was coping with the loss, suddenly I would see something or a thought would trigger a memory, and the hurt would flood right back in. Slowly, I learned not to try to understand it but to accept that the pain would never escape me completely. It would always be there, and at times it would surface, even when I least expected it.

Perhaps, like many couples, we should have kept the pregnancy a complete secret. It may have been the more sensible approach, but it would have been a much lonelier journey through both the happiness and the grief.

I did wonder how our friends and family felt about dealing with the aftermath of our loss. The pressure of providing words of comfort does not always come easy to some, and whilst it selfishly helped me to talk about the grief we were experiencing, something I desperately needed, perhaps it created unease for others? What I did know was that I needed that love and support, in whichever form it was offered. Whilst I perhaps didn't show my true appreciation at the time, it was the knowledge that I had people to lean on that helped me through to the other side of this grief.

# THE WHY

It was a natural question to ask when things went wrong. *Why? Why me? Why does this happen at all?* Unfortunately, there were no real answers to those questions. Mother Nature had the control, and it was her decision to rip away my dreams of motherhood. Could I have done something differently to change this fate? I would never truly know. All I knew was that it just felt so cruel and unfair.

Although I would never wish this fate on anyone else, there were times when I looked at other pregnant women and felt a little envious. Would I want them to experience even a moment of this grief? Never! But, it was a completely natural reaction for someone like me, and I found myself wondering why I hit the unlucky jackpot on the statistics front. I couldn't comprehend and accept that the odds were truly working against me.

I looked at my lifestyle, my age, my habits, and I wondered, *what if?* Was there anything I could change to help me beat these odds? It had almost become a desperation as I scoured the countless books, sites, and other sources of information to help me understand my position and my future chances of successfully conceiving and carrying a child. Yet nothing I have found gave me the answers I was seeking, and I was left with just a hanging doubt that there was that one thing that could have changed it all. What that was, I may never truly know . . .

It was hard not to feel that this situation was hopeless, and I wondered how I could possibly put myself through it all again without any further answers. I had to stop myself from questioning it all, avoiding the paranoia that constantly filtered into my own psyche. I forced myself to think positively and to hope that the next time we would find different odds.

As I slowly healed through the months, I had to stop myself from imagining where I would have be in my last pregnancy, had it been viable. I watched other women with their rounded bellies, and I wondered how I would have coped as the months progressed and my stomach swelled with a growing baby inside. I wondered what type of labour I would have experienced or even what our baby's gender would have been. There were so many unknowns, as it was all too early to tell. Our baby wasn't yet a fetus, but it was a life that was taken away well before its time.

I had to focus all of my will power to stop myself from over thinking the "why." I could not answer these questions myself; it would help nothing, and I was certainly not an expert in the field of medical science. Perhaps there was an answer out there, and I needed to pursue that answer, but through the right channels.

Perhaps the answer was this: It was all just unfortunate luck. It didn't give me any sense of closure, but it did help me have some hope that one day, that luck would turn. Why? If I didn't believe that, I might as well give up this dream of motherhood entirely.

# *THE OPTIONS*

Months after our most recent loss, it still hurt, but it was more of a numb, painful reminder of what could have been rather than the constant pain of grief that I felt immediately after. My body was back to normal, not pregnant. However, my mind was now open to what could be in our future if we explored our options once again.

In contemplating our next steps, thoughts started whirring through my mind. *Do we just start as we did before? What should we do differently? What happens next?* There were so many questions, and I was certainly not taking this decision lightly. To try again, and fail, well, that's something I would never really be prepared for. Then again, you can never prepare for that.

There was also that stark reminder that it wasn't just me in this game. I felt the physical side of the loss, but my husband had to watch my pain whilst also dealing with his own grief and the uncertainty around our future as parents. I had to consider both of us if we were to try again.

Where to start was the first and most important question. We had discussed our options at great length; we had even considered adoption as an alternative route, but there was something still unfinished in our pregnancy journey. We had to continue this quest to conceive successfully and carry a baby to full term.

I made an appointment with my doctor, hoping to seek out some more answers. Alas, I wasn't told anything that I couldn't find myself on the Internet. There were numerous tests we could undergo, but we were still walking blindly in all directions, trying to find a way out of this dark tunnel. There was no guarantee of answers, and that felt more frustrating than anything else. We could put my body through different courses of medication and examinations, spending time and money when we may never really know the true cause of our loss. There was no magic wand or specialist guru who could give us the real answer we needed.

The only common denominator in all our consultations was my age; at thirty-eight, I was just two years short of forty. It seemed like I was been constantly reminded that I would be a mature-age parent, and that I faced a high risk that the quality of my eggs may have a bearing on my ability to sustain a successful pregnancy. Although it was a risk factor, there was no real evidence to suggest my age was the reason my pregnancies failed; it was all just another game of odds. My doctor assured me that each egg is different, and perhaps not all my eggs are "bad," and I could likely become pregnant next time with a good egg.

This was just another factor that was completely out of my control. I could not stop time, and I certainly couldn't control Mother Nature's decision as to when and if I will fall pregnant again. In many ways I felt like I was spinning a roulette wheel on my chances of becoming a mother.

There was one question in particular that continued to surface as I faced each hiccup or setback. *How many losses are too many?* I found myself struggling to breathe sometimes with the mere thought that my quest to become a mother may never be fulfilled. *What will I do if I cannot fulfil this dream?* That thought alone kept me up night after night.

Once my body settled physically, and I felt ready to start trying again, I had to remind myself that I couldn't just rush into this without more thought. I felt that I needed to seriously think though my options for the future. I could not walk into this again blindly, and perhaps I felt I needed to be doing something, anything, that might feel different to the last time. I needed to have a plan of action, a way forward, or any assurance that this wouldn't happen again. Yet, I knew that I was looking for the impossible.

Like many couples, we also started to explore medical options, such as IVF. However, as I fell pregnant naturally quite easily, I was unsure what additional guarantees I could be given if we were to pursue this path. If it truly was the quality of my eggs and my age, I was told that the odds in our favour were still limited. Just the thought of experiencing another loss indicated that perhaps we needed a little more time before really deciding to move forward again.

The reality was, rushing straight into another pregnancy was not going to help me feel better about our past miscarriages. In fact, I wondered if it could potentially exacerbate a new set of anxieties, with no answers and just the looming thought of yet another potential loss.

We would certainly try again in the future; I was still determined to become a mother. However, there was so much more to consider in walking back down that path once again. I needed to ensure that I had the emotional and physical strength to endure whatever the fate of our next pregnancy may be. Balancing that, I could not really afford to wait too long, as my impending age barrier seemed to drive a higher risk on any future pregnancies. I felt that I was in a no-win situation either way.

I needed to force myself to breath, slow down, and refocus this energy towards healing and maintaining a positive mind-set. This was the time to remind myself what was truly important to me, myself, my sanity, my relationship with my husband, and the loved ones who have constantly rallied around me.

I was determined to prevail on this journey, but I could not do it all by myself.

# THE HOPE

Whether it is one miscarriage or many, starting over again, and getting back on that "trying to conceive" cycle, is such an incredibly daunting concept to come to terms with.

As I now consider my options, I do feel that all of my initial energy and enthusiasm that I had thrown into this journey at the very start, now feels slightly jaded. I wonder how long it will take to actually fall pregnant again, and when it does, I wonder how I will cope with being pregnant once again. I understand that it is all in my mind-set, and I need to ensure that my recharge battery is set into full-speed action. It's all or nothing, and I have to believe that our chances are strong, or else it's not worth even starting this journey once again.

If we want to continue down this road, and remain hopeful for a future which will involve children, we must start again. The fear of going through another miscarriage will always haunt me, but the dream of being a mother is so much stronger, that is what gives me the strength to keep pushing forward. Having considered our options in full, I know that I am not yet ready to stop this journey; I am in charge of my own emotions and my body, and there is a constant voice inside my heart that tells me that our time will come. That is the hope I need to hold on to, to keep me strong.

I can accept now that there are no absolute guarantees, yet despite that, I will continue to hold on to hope, dreaming of that day when I finally hold my own newborn baby in my arms.

I am constantly reminding myself that I cannot control my destiny and that this path towards motherhood may still be a little bumpy, and we may face more obstacles on the way. Perhaps it may lead to another destination, one that I had not expected. In the end, it is all a journey, and like many women in my situation, this one has not been an easy road to travel.

Right now, I can't see where the road ahead leads, but I can only keep moving forward, taking one step at a time, and facing each obstacle along the way with determination. Needless to say, I still believe that there is hope for me yet and that Mother Nature will eventually give in, offer some leniency and give me the child that I so desire.

I am ready to face the eye of the storm once more. I have prepared myself to battle the uncertainty it will force upon me, enduring its cruel wind and the sting of the rain. I have suffered through the damage of this storm and my memories are haunted by its pain and torment. Nevertheless, I am confident that with time, as the skies clear and the sun shines through, I will see the beautiful colours of a rainbow before me. That is the hope I need for a new tomorrow, a new beginning.

# THE LAST WORD

This is my story; well, it is just one of them. Like many women, I have several stories surrounding my quest to become a mother, and as I face each new chapter on this journey, I am faced with choices. I can choose to let the obstacles and roadblocks stop me, or I can choose to push forward and keep looking ahead.

In writing my story and sharing my experience with miscarriage, I have discovered many women who have also experienced a similar loss; some have had even tougher roads to travel, others are just starting their journey. The subject of miscarriage is starting to become less taboo in society, and yet in many ways the awkwardness still exists.

There have been instances, in social conversations where I am often asked when I plan to start a family. Even today, there is a expectation that most married couples will have children, as well as a naivety around the struggles that are often faced when trying to achieve this dream. Many times I have confronted these questions directly, sharing my struggles with infertility and miscarriage, and surprisingly the conversation suddenly turns very quiet with muffled apologies.

Perhaps I should remain silent on the issue, feign an excuse to save other's embarrassment? But why?

Personally, talking about my experiences and writing my story has helped me, allowing me to release my pain and connect with others, whether they have been down this road or not. I have met many brave, wonderful women who have given me hope and sometimes the strength I needed when I felt I was falling downwards.

My story is different to your story, and we all cope with loss and grief in distinct and separate ways. Many of the choices I have made on this journey, others would perhaps choose a different route.

Perhaps if I had my time over I may have chosen differently, however, I cannot dwell on regrets or "what ifs"; nor can I change the past. The only thing I can do is focus on the future, look ahead, not back, and allow myself to believe in tomorrow.

# ABOUT THE AUTHOR

Rachel McGrath grew up by the seaside in Queensland, Australia, where she studied business, before moving to the United Kingdom in her early thirties. She currently lives just north of London in Hertfordshire, where she met and married her husband.

Rachel has always had a passion for writing both fiction and non-fiction. Since her early teens, she has created many short stories as well as smaller pieces that have never been published.

Rachel published her first book in early 2015, **Finding the Rainbow**, an award winning memoir capturing her struggle to conceive and carry a child.

Rachel has also published several children's fiction stories and continues to work on further writing projects.

# *FINDING THE RAINBOW*

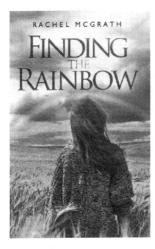

Finding the Rainbow is the award winning, fascinating and honest insight into a world that most would find difficult to understand, and many would be quietly thankful not to need to. McGrath tells the story of her battle to conceive and carry a baby, with unrestricted honesty, leaving the reader in no doubt as to her thoughts and feelings, and the courageousness with which she deals with a very difficult period in her and her husband's lives. This emotive account draws attention to some of the otherwise unknown aspects of infertility and miscarriage, whilst still leaving room for humour, happiness and philosophy. The first book for Rachel McGrath, she writes about her battle with her body, her mind and the health service, whilst showing an incredible amount of inner strength, elegance and poise.

Please enjoy a sample chapter from *Finding the Rainbow:*

*We were married almost a year when we finally decided to 'try' to have a baby. It seemed like the 'right' thing to do, and we were in no hurry. I guess we had assumed this would be a lot easier. Up until then, I was on the pill, and had been for many years. For me, I was going to stop taking the pill one day and voila, baby would appear nine months later... Right? Wrong! I had no idea how this would work, but I had this fantastical notion that it just would.*

*We left for our dream holiday to the Maldives, and I had left that contraceptive pill packet at home, throwing chance to the wind, believing for sure that we would be pregnant and telling our friends and family the exciting news on return from holiday. Naïve you say? I certainly was!*

*We naturally had many opportunities on this holiday to make it happen, but not surprisingly my period arrived shortly after we returned from holiday. To be honest, I really didn't know much about the pregnancy journey, and I was thinking that it was potentially several bouts of good sex, and the timing and results would then just magically work themselves out.*

*I had heard so many stories of women who 'accidently' fall pregnant, so I assumed my own experience would be a piece of cake. However, I quickly realised that more information was needed on how this 'trying to conceive' notion worked. Unbeknown to me this was the world I had avoided for many years, as my intention was always 'not to get pregnant', and at this point in time, I had to do a complete about face, landing smack bang into our new focus – get pregnant quick! I was, after all, thirty-six and to me time was definitely running out!*

*Whilst it was still all about enjoying the baby-making sex, which of course is the fun part, it was now also about timing, tests, symptoms, positions, and sometimes just watching a calendar month on month, and then waiting for the next cycle. Suddenly there was the realisation that having a baby is pretty serious business, life changing and something we couldn't just be frivolous about. The entire process made me more appreciative of the responsibilities and commitment that beheld parenthood, and what it would really mean to be a parent one day, hopefully.*

Purchase **Finding the Rainbow** on Amazon, Barnes and Noble and all other online retailers.

www.findingtherainbow.net

# Other Publications by **RACHEL McGRATH**

FINDING THE RAINBOW

DARK & TWISTY: A Twisted Anthology of
Short Stories

MUD ON YOUR FACE

GRIMWALD'S EVIL PLAN (Coming Soon)

WONDERFUL WORLD OF WILLOW

COCO THE CRAZY PUP

94975443R00047

Made in the USA
San Bernardino, CA
14 November 2018